THE
ART OF
BREATHING

How to Become at Peace
with Yourself and the World

Danny Penman, PhD

Foreword by Jon Kabat-Zinn
Afterword by Mark Williams

HAMPTON ROADS

Cover design by Kathryn Sky-Peck

Book design by Steve Wells

Hampton Roads Publishing Company, Inc.

Charlottesville, VA 22906

Distributed by Red Wheel/Weiser, LLC

www.redwheelweiser.com

ISBN: 978-1-64297-042-5

Library of Congress Cataloging-in-Publication Data available upon request.

Library of Congress Control Number: 2017958237

Printed in Canada

MAR

10 9 8 7 6 5 4 3 2 1

Dedicated to my wife Bella
and our two boisterous kids
Sasha and Luka.

CONTENTS

Download meditations from www.franticworld.com/breathing

FOREWORD

Among all the dimensions of life we take for granted
or ignore, and there are many, breathing is among the
closest to us and the most fundamental. We are always
only one breath away from not being able to keep the
mystery of this universe comprising trillions of human
cells* that we somehow think of as "me" alive. The entire
constellation miraculously and unceasingly takes care of
itself through breathing, over seconds, minutes, hours,
days, weeks, months, years, and decades. What a gift.
What an opportunity—if only we could wake up to it.
And that is what mindfulness, or what we might call
openhearted wakefulness is all about . . . pure awareness,
boundless, centerless, and already yours. Perhaps our
awareness is the most unique characteristic of our
humanity—the final common pathway of what makes
us who we are and might be, both as a species and as
individuals.

*The official estimate is in the 37 trillion range at the moment, and that is not counting the approximately equal
number of bacteria (known collectively as the microbiome) living in our digestive tract and all over the body.
Apparently the number of cells in the human body is hugely larger than the estimated number of galaxies in the
entire universe by about 800 billion.

When we think of the breath at all, we routinely think of it as "my breath." We say things like "I am breathing," but frankly, if it were up to us to keep the breathing going, we would have died a long time ago, especially in this age of perpetual self-distraction. A text, an e-mail, a thought: DEAD. So whoever we think we are when we deploy those singular personal pronouns "I," "me," or "mine," "we" are not allowed anywhere near ultimate control of the brain stem, the phrenic nerve, and the diaphragm's ongoing collaboration to keep this universe we call "me" alive. We are simply not reliable enough for the job. And that's a good thing, because it frees us up for other kinds of adventures, especially taking full advantage of the life that is ours to live while the breath is still mysteriously moving in and out.

All this is to say that we can intentionally befriend the breath to great advantage. And that is what Danny Penman's beautifully tactile and invitingly pleasing and uplifting gift to us is all about. We can cultivate exquisite intimacy with the breath, which in turn, cultivates intimacy with life itself, with our body, our mind, our thoughts, our emotions, our imagination, our creativity, our beauty. Ultimately, it puts us in touch with our relationality to everything, outwardly as well as inwardly, including our embeddedness in the social and the natural worlds, in a word, with who and what we are, more akin to pure awareness than anything else. After all, we are collectively known as Homo sapiens sapiens, the species that is aware and knows that it is aware.

This book is an exquisitely accessible and welcoming door into that entire universe. Enter, enter, enter and ultimately befriend yourself in your fullness as part of a much larger whole.

—Jon Kabat-Zinn

author of *Full Catastrophe Living*,
Professor of Medicine Emeritus at the University of
Massachusetts Medical School and founder of its Center for
Mindfulness in Medicine, Health Care, and Society

one: IN THE BEGINNING

Six paragliders are circling like eagles on powerful currents of rising air. Far below, a cluster of children gaze with open mouths as the giant parachutes dive and swoosh silently above their heads.

Then, suddenly, something starts to go wrong.

One of the paragliders is hit by a powerful gust of wind, turning the canopy inside out. The pilot starts spinning, spiraling like a sycamore seed toward the earth.

After an eternity, the young man smashes into the hillside. He lies face down on the ground. Broken.

But he is alive. After a moment of stunned silence, he begins screaming in agony. It will be at least thirty minutes before the paramedics arrive. And another hour to reach the hospital.

Alone, he knows that
he can't afford to lose
consciousness in case he
never again awakens. So
he begins forcing himself
to breathe.

Slowly. Deeply. With a
supreme effort of will,
he focuses his mind
away from his broken
body and onto his
breath. In. Out.

Inch by inch, the agony
recedes. Before, finally,
he reaches a state of calm
tranquility.

Of pure mindfulness.

I was the young
man who crashed
his paraglider.

The
art of
breathing
saved
my life.

For thousands of years, people have used the art of breathing for equally profound effects on the mind and body.

Some have used it for relief from chronic pain. Many more to cope with anxiety, stress and depression. Some claim it led to spiritual enlightenment.

But I'm as spiritual as a housebrick . . .

. . . so I use it to help me appreciate the bittersweet beauty of everyday life.

Your breath is the greatest asset you have. It's naturally meditative and always with you. It reflects your most powerful emotions and allows you to either soothe or harness them. It helps you to feel solid, whole, and in complete control of your life while grounding you in the present moment, clarifying the mind, and unshackling your instincts.

The art of breathing kindles a sense of wonder, awe, and curiosity—the very foundations of a happier and more meaningful life.

It grants you the courage to accept yourself with all of your faults and failings. To treat yourself with the kindness, empathy and compassion that you truly need, and helps you to look outward and embrace the world.

When you've
mastered the art
of breathing,
you will finally
be at peace with
yourself and the
world.

two: **BREATHING**

As long as you are breathing, there is more right with you than wrong with you.—*Jon Kabat-Zinn*

It all begins with your very first breath . . .

Just after being born, imperceptibly at first, but with slowly building momentum, your tiny lungs began to inflate.

Nestling in your mother's arms, you began learning how to breathe. It wasn't easy.

A baby's breathing isn't naturally rhythmic. Babies breathe only when they need to, often with terrifyingly long gaps between breaths, not with a natural fluid motion.

As the weeks passed into months, your breathing developed its own natural rhythm. But, even now, you can soak up the rhythms of another's breath.

Lovers' breaths are entwined. Crowds breathe in harmony. Even the breaths of our pets can become entrained with ours.

None of us are separate.

Although it feels stubbornly so.

You breathe 22,000 times a day. How many are you aware of?

REMEMBERING TO BREATHE

Your breathing is so ordinary, so mundane, that its true significance can easily pass you by.

Lie flat on the ground with a cushion under your head. Place your hands on your stomach. Feel them rise and fall as you breathe in . . . and out.

As the breath waxes and wanes, the abdominal organs rise and fall by 1½ to 2 inches. This pumps oxygen and nutrient-rich fluids through the lymphatic system, flushing out toxins. The physical movement of the breath in the body also massages the liver, kidneys, intestines, joints of the spine, indeed everything, so they're kept healthy, supple, and well lubricated.

The breath is life . . .

. . . on countless levels.

Your breathing both reflects and amplifies your emotions

Momentary stress causes the body to tense and you begin to breathe a little more shallowly. A shallow breath lowers oxygen levels in the blood, which the brain senses as stress.

Breathing becomes a little quicker and shallower. Oxygen levels fall a little more.

The heart begins to race. The brain feels a little more stressed.

IT'S A VICIOUS CYCLE

But there is an alternative . . .

A gently rising and falling breath stimulates the parasympathetic nervous system.

You begin to relax.

These calm negative thoughts, feelings and emotions so you begin to breathe a little more slowly and deeply.

Soothing hormones flow through the body.

IT'S A VIRTUOUS CYCLE

BREATHE
IN

BREATHE
OUT

When in doubt, breathe out.

Most of us breathe incorrectly.

Breathing relies on the big, powerful muscles of the diaphragm, the abdomen and the intercostal muscles that lie between the ribs. It is helped along by the smaller secondary muscles of the neck, shoulders, and upper ribs.

When you are upset, anxious or stressed, the abdomen tenses and prevents the big primary muscles from working. Instead, they begin tugging against each other, leaving the secondary muscles to do all the work. But the secondary muscles are only designed to shoulder 20 percent of the burden, so they become stressed.

If this continues, it can lead to chronic tension in the shoulders and neck, to headaches and fatigue, and to increasingly shallower breathing.

It really is as simple as breathing . . .

To breathe correctly, all you need to do is set your breath
free. Mindfully submit to its natural rhythm. Feel the
air as it flows in and out of your body. Allow yourself to
relax into the breath's fluidity.

Feel your shoulders loosen and unfurl. Close your eyes
(if you want to) and feel the ground beneath your feet.

If you feel anxious, distressed, unhappy, or exhausted,
then begin to consciously breathe in and out.

Take a long, deep breath while
counting slowly to 5 in your mind.
Pause for a moment. Then breathe
out while counting to 7.

You can alter the speed of the counting to reflect the
unique rhythm of your breath. Try not to rush things.

Repeat this 5/7 breathing until you feel
more solid, whole, and in control. You can
come back to it as often as you like.

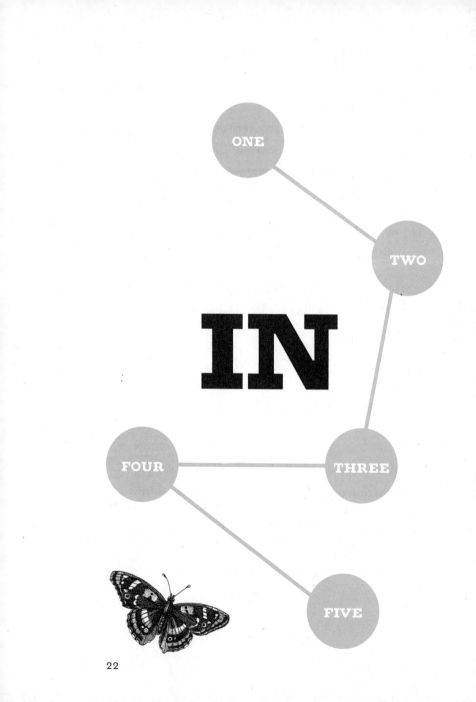

ONE

TWO

IN

FOUR

THREE

FIVE

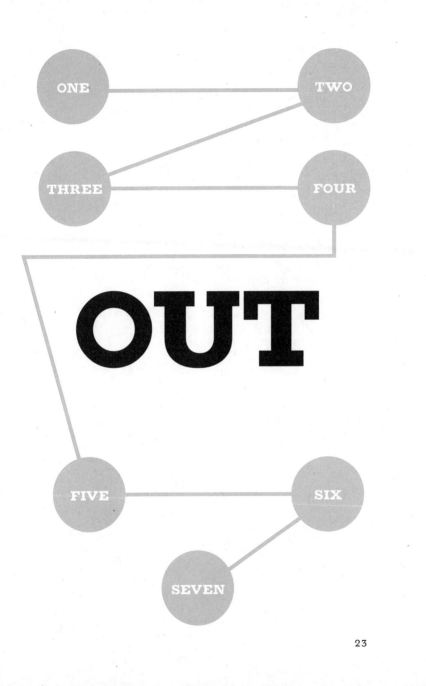

ONE   TWO
THREE   FOUR

OUT

FIVE   SIX
SEVEN

three: MINDFULNESS

The art of breathing lies in paying attention to your breath in a very special way. It's the heart of mindfulness and as old as meditation itself. You can learn the basics in just a few minutes . . .

. . . but mastering the art of breathing takes somewhat longer.

Breathing meditations are very simple but people often make them difficult and complicated.

Firstly, meditating in the lotus position is very uncomfortable. You can't meditate if you're not comfortable. Take a deep breath . . .

. . . and ask why the chair was invented.

Secondly, you don't need any equipment, mantras, incense, fancy bells, apps, or even a quiet room.

In fact, all you
need is:

a Chair
a Body
some Air
your Mind
that's It.

BREATHING MEDITATION

Sit on a straight-backed chair. Place your feet flat on the floor (with your spine one inch from the back of the chair). Be comfortable (with a relaxed but straight back). Place your hands loosely in your lap.

Close your eyes.

Focus your mind on your breath as it flows in and out. Feel the sensations the air makes as it flows in through your mouth or nose and into your lungs. Feel the rising and falling of your chest and stomach.

Where are the strongest feelings? Nose, mouth, throat, stomach, chest, shoulders? Pay attention and explore the feelings, especially the way they rise and fall. Don't try to alter them in any way or expect anything special to happen.

When your mind wanders,
bring it back to your breath.
Be kind to yourself. Minds
wander. It's what they do.
Realizing that your mind
has wandered and bringing
it back to your breath *is* the
meditation. It's a little moment
of mindfulness.

Your mind may eventually become
calm for a little while, or filled with
thoughts or feelings such as anger,
stress, or love. These may be fleeting.
See them as clouds in the sky (simply
watch them drift past). Try not to
change anything. Gently return your
awareness back to the sensations of
breathing again and again.

After five minutes (or longer if you can manage) gently open your eyes and take in what you can see, hear, feel, and smell.

Repeat twice a day.

A person whose mind isn't wandering, isn't meditating.

Did you feel restless and uncomfortable? Discover a few aches and pains? Perhaps there was a long list of things that needed doing RIGHT NOW, THIS MINUTE.

Maybe you had wild swings of energy. One moment you were bubbling with enthusiasm, then suddenly . . . exhausted.

And the powerful emotions that swept you along— the frustrations and disappointments, the feelings of inadequacy followed by the bitter taste of defeat as yet again you realized that your mind had wandered away from your breath.

You probably felt that your mind was so chaotic you will never be able to focus for more than a few seconds at a time. What a mess . . .

This is normal.

It's your first lesson.

Minds
wander.
It's what
they do.

This leads to the central guiding
principle of mindfulness:
you cannot fail. Realizing that your
mind has wandered away from the
breath *is* the meditation.

It is a moment of mindfulness.

MINDFULNESS IS FULL CONSCIOUS AWARENESS.

It is paying full conscious attention to whatever thoughts, feelings and emotions are flowing through your mind, body, and breath without judging or criticizing them in any way.

It is being fully aware of whatever is happening in the present moment without being trapped in the past or worrying about the future.

It is living *in* the moment not *for* the moment.

MINDFULNESS
IS NOT
A RELIGION

Nor is it
"opting out"
or detaching
yourself from
the world.

It's about
connecting
and embracing
life in all of its
chaotic beauty,
with all of
your faults and
foibles.

THE AIM OF MINDFULNESS IS NOT TO INTENTIONALLY CLEAR THE MIND OF THOUGHTS

It is to understand how the mind works. To see how it unwittingly ties itself in knots to create anxiety, stress, unhappiness, and exhaustion.

It teaches you to observe how your thoughts, feelings, and emotions rise and fall like waves on the sea.

And in the calm spaces in between lie moments of piercing insight.

YOU ARE NOT YOUR THOUGHTS. YOU ARE THE AWARENESS THAT ALREADY KNOWS YOUR THOUGHTS ARE THOUGHTS, WITHOUT HAVING TO THINK IT.

It's a subtle distinction that's only perceived with practice.

Your thoughts are a running commentary on the world; a "best guess" of what's truly happening. Often, your thoughts will reflect the powerful emotional currents swirling through your mind, body, and breath.

Sometimes they are true, sometimes they are a frantic work in progress, sometimes they are wrong.

Mindfulness teaches you to take the long view, to put your thoughts, feelings, and emotions into a broader context.

And when you do so, your most frantic and distressing thoughts simply melt away of their own accord, leaving behind a calm, clear, insightful mind.

four: **HAPPINESS**

Happiness is fleeting whilst unhappiness lingers.

It's called the "Negativity Bias" and it's hardwired into the very core of our being. It skews perception and makes the world seem far harsher, bleaker, and more competitive than it actually is.

But life really is full of opportunities and pleasures.

It's just that the brain routinely tricks us into thinking otherwise. Luckily, we can redress the balance with the art of breathing.

It works like this:

Nature compels us to avoid threats and seek out resources. It's one of the driving forces behind Natural Selection, but it comes with a powerful, inbuilt bias. Far better to avoid threats, and survive, even if it means we fail to gain any number of rewards.

Instinct encourages us to assume the worst, to err on the side of caution, to live in fear and hide in the background.

The Negativity Bias ensures that it takes five positive experiences to balance a single negative one of equal magnitude.

This is a little dispiriting.

But then again, Nature doesn't care if we're happy but she does take a keen interest in our survival.

That's the point of Natural Selection, after all.

Thankfully, we are conscious creatures, so we can restore the balance and gain a happier and more accurate picture of the world.

It's no more difficult than periodically tuning into the breath while paying attention to the little pleasures of daily life. It means noticing the sights, sounds, smells, and textures that surround you and soaking up the tastes and aromas of everything that you eat and drink.

It means giving your senses the attention they deserve while allowing them to intensify naturally.

And, while you do so, gently remind yourself that . . .

. . . most of life's difficulties are only half as bad as they appear, while the good things are two or three times as intense.

Fig.13.

Fig.9.

Fig.3.

Fig.10.

Fig.6.

Fig.8.

Fig.2.

Begin by
eating some
fruit.

FRUIT MEDITATION

Choose a type of fruit that you haven't eaten recently (or even better, one that you've never eaten before).

Ground yourself by focusing on the rise and fall of your breath for 20–30 seconds.

Look at the fruit. Let your eyes soak up everything you can see. Is it smooth, furry, rough, jagged, or shiny?

Inhale its smell.

Peel the fruit (if it's the kind that needs peeling).

Close your eyes.

Take a bite. How do your teeth feel as they slice through the fruit? Hold the fruit in your mouth for a while. How does it feel? Hard, slimy, stringy, crunchy, or mushy? Soak up the texture. What can you taste? Can you sense the different flavors? Sweet, sour, bitter, acidic? Your mind will wander. When you realize, gently bring it back to your breath for a few moments and then return to the fruit.

After a while, gently chew the fruit. Hold the mush in your mouth for a while. Swallow. How does it feel? Repeat with another bite. Then another, until you've almost finished.

Squash the remaining piece of fruit here:

How do you feel now? Why not bring this flavor of awareness to the rest of your day? ADAPT (and use for any other type of food or drink: soup, stew, vegetables, bread (or even chocolate, tea, or coffee).

five: CURIOSITY

It's impossible to be unhappy and curious at the same time.

BUT HABITS KILL CURIOSITY.

And around half of your life is ruled by habit.

They may streamline your life and free up time
and energy for you to do more useful and
interesting things.

But they can also become a trap . . . quite a vicious one.
Habits begin wearing grooves in the mind and become
hardwired into your brain.

One habit triggers the next, and the next, so that whole
chunks of your life are run on autopilot.
Unless you're careful, they'll
control almost every aspect of
your life, including your taste in
food, clothes, music, and even
your choice of partners.

Habits govern how you interact with everyone around you, how you solve problems, how you conjure up "new" ideas, and your entire approach to the world.

As Aristotle once said, "We are what we repeatedly do."

Habits can enhance limitations and trap you in negative states of mind. And the more often you criticize yourself, the easier it is to slip into the same habit the next time, and the next, and the next.

- What's up with me today?
- Why do I keep doing stupid things like this?
- Why can't I just do it?
- My life's a bit of a mess.
- I'm exhausted.

One thought triggers the next, and the next, in an endless downward spiral.

It's the sound of your inner critic—and it's always with you.

Your inner critic is the voice of the Negativity Bias. And you're ushering it along by habit.

But habits

aren't

destiny,

unless you

allow them

to be.

In fact, you can breathe them away.

Habits arise when your mind is elsewhere.

They dissolve when you mindfully bring your focus back to the present moment. Observe your habits often enough and their underlying neural patterns will wither away to leave behind a calmer, clearer, more insightful mind.

So, when you realize you've been snared by an unwanted habit, or feel trapped by your inner critic, or suffer from anxious, stressful, bleak, or otherwise negative thoughts . . .

. . . do something they'll really hate.

Take a few,
gentle, deep
breaths.
Feel the
ground
beneath
your feet . . .

Take a breathing space.... Adopt your usual meditation posture (or stand if you prefer). Gently close your eyes.

BREATHING SPACE MEDITATION

Step 1:
Arriving

Begin by noticing whatever is going on around you. Become aware of the space around you. Feel the ground beneath your feet.

What's going on in your mind and body right now? Briefly scan through your body and tune in to the most noticeable sensations. Don't try to change anything, simply feel the sensations.

Begin paying attention to the emotions flowing through your mind and body. Don't try to change anything, pay attention to their intensity and notice how they rise and fall.

What thoughts are around? Don't try to change anything. Simply observe them. Remember that thoughts are not facts.

Step 2:
Focusing

Shift your awareness to your breath.
Follow it all the way in and all the way
out for thirty seconds or so. Each time
your mind wanders, gently escort your
awareness back to your breath.

Step 3:
Expanding

Begin to broaden your awareness to include your whole body. Feel your whole body breathing for thirty seconds or so. If there are any areas of tension or discomfort, imagine breathing into them with a sense of warmth and kindness.

Then begin to progressively broaden your awareness to encompass the space around you. Gently open your eyes.

CURIOSITY KILLS HABITS.

Things to break and do . . .

Habits are the mind's sheepdogs. Set yourself free by unleashing your curiosity. Do as many of the following as you wish.

Whatever you do, do it consciously, with full awareness.

Be Curious. Be Energetic. Be Alive.

Spend thirty minutes less at work.

Sit at a different table or chair.

Pick up a new book to get lost in.

Watch the sky
for half an hour.

Take a
different
commute to
work.

Stop every two
hours and
consciously breathe.

Go to the seaside,
the countryside, the
mountains, or even
the local park.

Switch
supermarkets.

Eat something
you've never
eaten before.

six: **PLAYFULNESS**

You'll probably spend thirty-six minutes worrying today (most people do). Why not go outside and breathe instead?

When you were a child, the world was a magical place.
You'd go to the park and collect pinecones and flowers.
Birds inspired awe and dogs were mythical beasts.

You could hardly make it home without your pockets
becoming stuffed with twigs, stones, and other souvenirs.

Where did all that playful curiosity go?

nowhere

It's simply become paved over with expectations,
conditioning, and maybe a little shyness and cynicism.

It's time to breathe freely again.

escape from
your habits

SCAVENGER MEDITATION

You will need:
One shoebox (or something similar). Some paperclips. A snack (you mightn't be back in time for tea).
That's it.

Switch off your phone (you don't want to be distracted). Tuck your shoebox under your arm and walk outside, close your eyes and focus on the sensations of breathing. Feel the ground beneath your feet.

Walk to your nearest park or empty lot. Wander around, following idle curiosity.

What catches your eye? A pile of leaves? Fading flowers. Some rubbish? If you feel drawn to something in particular, how does it affect your breath? Does your heart speed up? Do you feel excited? Feel the years falling away.

If something looks especially interesting, touch it or pick it up. Peer at all of its nooks and crannies (you're a child, remember). What does it feel like? Rough, smooth, ridged, soft, slimy, or slippery? Soak up the textures. Smell it. Fresh, musty, earthy, or stinky? Use all of your senses to explore what you find; you can even listen to it (remember the sound of the sea in a seashell?).

Let the scavenging begin; collect five objects and put them in your shoebox. It doesn't matter what they are, they just need to resonate with you in some way, whether they be twigs, petals, coins, or chips bags.

Either now or later, take your objects and spread them out. What's their story? If you found a man-made object, what was it originally used for? Where was it made? Who made it? Can you imagine what their life was like? How did it reach the park or empty lot?

For a natural item, where did it grow? Which wildlife relied on it for food, shelter or protection? Spend some time engaging with each object in this fashion and placing it into a wider context.

Close your eyes. Breathe. Imagine the web of connections binding us all together. Humanity and nature. Nature and humanity.

Breathe. Be playful. Stay curious. Paperclip something
you found on your scavenging trip to this page. It could
be a rose petal, a bus ticket, or a leaf. The choice is yours,
but make it consciously.

Fig. 3.

Fig. 9.

Fig. 10.

Fig. 8.

Fig. 6.

seven: **AWARENESS**

All that is solid melts into air. *

* Apologies to Marx and Engels (they'd probably think meditation is
a "capitalist running-dog conspiracy." It isn't, in case you were wondering.)

Thoughts, feelings, and
emotions are created
by the body as much as
the brain. Even logic
and rationality are
profoundly influenced
by the body.

It ensures that you see the world as a reflection of yourself—rather than as objective reality.

Fancy a nice cup of tea?

If you want someone to like and trust you, give them a warm drink. Empathy and trust are warm.

If you're seeking a more masculine aura, give them something hard to hold. Masculine is hard.
If you want something to appear more valuable, make it heavy. Valuable is heavy.

Embodied cognition is the body's shorthand. It summarizes and simplifies so you can make quick decisions in a complex and rapidly changing world.

Unluckily, embodied cognition can lock you into negative spirals that lead to anxiety, stress, unhappiness, and exhaustion.

A fleeting moment of stress creates tension in the body. The brain senses this physical tension and interprets it as stress. The body tenses a little more, breathing becomes a little shallower. The brain feels a little more stressed.

It's a downward spiral.

The same holds true for many other states of mind. The mind is reflected in the body—and the body in the mind. So states of mind and body can all feed back off each other in complex and unexpected ways.

When you
think about it,
it's amazing that
we're as sane and
well balanced as
we are.

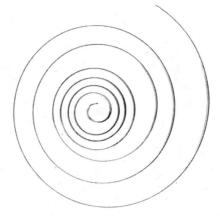

But, luckily, we have this magical
dimension of being human called
consciousness.

It allows you to see the interconnections between your
mind and body, and releases you from negative and
reactive states of mind.

So instead you can learn to *respond* rather than react.

And such awareness

is only ever a

single breath away.

STOP
BREATHE

Mindful breathing teaches you that your most powerful states of mind are reflected in the body as physical sensations.

Be aware of these sensations. Each one is a message.

If you ignore them or suppress them, then they will become ever more insistent and distressing until you can resist them no longer.

It's one of the most powerful sources of unhappiness and distress.

But there is an alternative.

If you consciously listen to these messages by actively feeling them in your body, then something miraculous can happen. You'll realize that they rise and fall like the waves on the sea or your breath in your body.

And before long they'll begin to melt away of their own accord, leaving behind a calmer, happier, and more insightful mind.

Listen to
your body.

Listen
to your
breathing.

Become aware of your stress and watch it dissolve. Begin by tuning in to your breath. Feel its rise and fall. After a minute or so, begin paying attention to your body and locate where your unpleasant feelings or emotions have taken root.

Stress might be found as tightness in your chest, shoulders, or neck. Anxiety as twitchiness in your hands, legs, or stomach. Unhappiness as heaviness in your face. It doesn't matter where they are to be found, simply tune in to them and explore how they feel.

Do the sensations feel "tight," painful, or achy? Or perhaps "loose," exciting, weak, or fleeting? It doesn't matter how they feel. Simply explore what you find.

When you realize that your mind has wandered, gently refocus your awareness back on the breath for a few moments, then begin exploring the physical feelings once again.

Notice how they rise and fall. Consciously feel them for a minute or so before mentally breathing into them. With each breath, does their intensity rise before falling away again? Notice how their patterns begin to change and then start to dissolve.

After a minute or so (or for longer if you can) broaden your awareness to encompass the rest of your body. Then broader still, to include your surroundings. What can you hear, feel, smell, or even taste? Gently open your eyes.

Repeat this practice whenever unpleasant thoughts, feelings, or emotions arise.

Mindfulness is
the observation
and acceptance of
your wandering
thoughts.

Whatever happens,
always remember
that you cannot fail
at meditation.

MINDFULNESS IS OBSERVATION WITHOUT CRITICISM.

When you are meditating, try not to set yourself a definite goal, such as clearing your mind of thoughts or aiming to become happier or more peaceful or content.

These are often happy by-products of meditation. But if you aim for them, you will miss.

It may seem like an annoying paradox, but it is also true.

When you meditate, you find what you find.

eight: **INSIGHTFULNESS**

IN

Everything breathes . . . even the ground beneath
your feet and the stars above your head.

Our planet begins drawing her breath in May.

For months, global oxygen levels have been falling
and carbon dioxide concentrations rising.

Then something miraculous happens—the sun
crosses an invisible threshold, triggering the vast forests
and grasslands of the Northern Hemisphere to set leaf
and bloom.

As they turn green and photosynthesize, they start
sucking unimaginable quantities of carbon dioxide
out from the atmosphere and releasing oxygen as
a by-product.

It begins almost overnight and accelerates rapidly. The northern Spring races forth at forty-five miles a day and then turns into summer.

The Earth's in-breath lasts for five months.

There's a brief pause.

Before autumn arrives and winter rushes in. Leaves begin to fall and grass to wither. As they break down, they consume oxygen and return vast quantities of carbon dioxide to the atmosphere.*

* These cyclical atmospheric changes are driven largely by the vast temperate forests and grasslands of the Northern Hemisphere. Take a look at this beautiful NASA video via *www.franticworld.com/breathing*

OUT

Elements of every breath you take
have been breathed by every person
in history.

Einstein, Shakespeare, Leonardo da Vinci.

Molecules from those breaths are still swirling
through the air, being inhaled and exhaled, becoming
incorporated into our bodies, turned into flesh and
bone, into other animals, plants, and rocks.

Wisps of those breaths first arose billions of years ago,
inside exploding stars.

Stars draw their first breath when vast swirling clouds of hydrogen in deep space begin to condense. They become hotter, denser, until . . .

. . . the immense heat and pressure inside the stars foment a vast, uncontrollable, run-away nuclear reaction that continues for billions of years.

The stars twinkle and shine.

A sudden outbreath . . .

The star explodes in a supernova, showering the galaxy
with the elements needed for planets to form,
for an atmosphere to be created, and for life to evolve.

Every molecule of the air you breathe, every atom in
your body was born inside an exploding star billions of
years ago.

You needn't be a mystic to have mystical moments . . .

. . . you just need a basic knowledge of physics.

TIME TO TAKE A BREATHER...

Go outside on a starry night. Take off your shoes and socks. Feel the ground beneath your feet.

Look upward.

Breathe.

See the stars streaming off into infinity in every direction. Not just unimaginably big but true, never-ending, ever-expanding infinity.

Focus on your breath as it flows in and out. Feel the soles of your feet touching the ground, the cool night air washing over you.

Feel the stillness, the expectation, infinity itself . . .

Look at the stars as they twinkle. Those twinkles may have taken billions of years to reach you.

Breathe.

Love, love
the arriving
of the light . . .

Breathe.

Our universe first appeared as a "singularity": a point of infinite energy and density that erupted out of nothingness.

A fluctuation in emptiness.

Space and time tore out from this at near-infinite speed.

One "moment" there was nothing. The next, everything.

An exhalation, if you like.

The universe will begin its end when space and time cease to expand.

Everything will pause for a while.

And then begin racing back to a singularity at an ever accelerating pace.

An inhalation, if you will.

For centuries, people have prepared
their mind with a very special breathing
meditation before contemplating
such ideas.

The quality of mind it engenders has countless other
benefits too.

It enhances creativity and clarity of thought while
promoting a sense of peace and well-being. It encourages
a sense of wonder, of awe, of curiosity—the foundations
of a happier and more meaningful life.

It soothes the inner critic and allows your true self
to bubble through to the surface. It will give you the
courage to accept yourself with all of your faults and
failings. To treat yourself with the kindness, empathy,
and compassion that you truly need . . . so you can look
outward and embrace the world.

And when you do this . . .

. . . you'll discover the secret to living mindfully.

INSIGHT MEDITATION

Sit.

Close your eyes and tune into the world around you, becoming aware of the space around you. You might hear some noise. . . . Whatever is there, pay attention to the sounds for a few moments.

Begin building up a picture of how your body feels, beginning with your feet. Pay attention to both feet simultaneously for a few moments. Tune into the sensations, then move your attention to the ankles . . . the lower legs . . . knees . . . upper legs . . . hips and pelvis . . .

Take your time. There's no rush.

Move your attention
to both hands . . .
arms . . . shoulders . . .
neck . . . head . . . face
. . . nose . . . and lips.

Soak
everything up,
in turn, over a
minute or so.

Pay attention to the
movement of your breath
in your body—follow it all
the way in . . . and all the
way out. Don't try to change
anything, just feel its natural,
flowing rhythm.

When you realize that your
mind has wandered, watch the
thoughts themselves. It doesn't
matter whether they're in the
form of words or pictures, simply
pay attention for a few moments
and then return to the breath.

After a couple of minutes, shift your awareness to any thoughts or emotions passing through your mind.

These thoughts and emotions—and the gaps in between them—will now become the focus of the meditation.

Don't force any thoughts to appear in your mind, simply wait patiently for them to arrive. Let the mind be completely free . . . free from any control or expectation.

Try to become aware of the moment that thoughts first appear, then watch them for a few moments. Notice how they rise and fall; how one thought triggers the next and the next.

Notice how thoughts tend to melt away when you stop reacting to them, when you stop judging or criticizing them.

Notice what happens when your thoughts momentarily stop . . . try to gain a sense of what it feels like . . . try to gain a sense of what the absence of thoughts feels like.

It might feel like a place of pure tranquility or it might feel like an emptiness or perhaps of something vast just beyond your grasp. Whatever it seems like, simply wait as if you're sitting on the edge of a vast pool. Waiting. Patiently . . .

After a while you'll realize that your mind has wandered away with itself again. When you do so, gently shift your attention back to the breath, and after a few breaths begin waiting patiently for another thought or emotion to appear.

You may run through this cycle of mind wandering and refocusing countless times. It doesn't matter. What matters is paying attention to your mind with all of its toings and froings.

Checking out.

After ten minutes or so, gradually begin to shift your attention to the world around you, becoming aware of the space around you. Open your eyes. Begin to move. See if you can maintain the essence of this clear-sighted awareness as you move through your day.

The Insight Meditation works best if you practice regularly. Ten or twenty minutes a day, four or five days a week is sufficient.

At the beginning of this book
you took a breath, maybe your first
conscious breath in years and
one of the most important breaths
you've ever taken.

Take a few moments to reflect
about how far you've come and
how the journey has already begun
to transform your life.

The art of breathing lies in having
the courage to let go. To let go and
allow your breath to breathe itself.
And when you do this, something
miraculous begins to happen, life
begins to live through you.

You become quicker to laugh and slower to anger; life becomes less frantic and exhausting, sleep more restful. You rediscover your sense of wonder, awe, and outright joy.

But most of all, you accept your imperfections with a warm smile rather than biting criticism.

Now breathe.

AFTERWORD

This is a gem of a book. Danny Penman brings together his skills as a teacher and writer and, with artist Steve Wells, creates beautiful images and word pictures. What you see on the page is nothing less than what your life might be if, for just a moment, you could slow down and notice your breath. Sounds so easy, doesn't it? As if you could do it with no effort at all. But Danny explains that the habits that send you rushing through each day are often so powerful that even the idea of taking a pause, of looking after yourself, rarely takes root. Instead, you live your life trapped in a hamster wheel of distraction, stress, and exhaustion, then feel guilty about how things have turned out.

This book says there is an alternative way to live your life, and it's right here. It speaks in a different voice—the quiet voice of the heart, inviting you to try an experiment that takes no more than a few minutes a day. As you've seen, it offers simple meditation practices that can bring you into another mode of being—more aware, less stressed, more compassionate, more alive—without having to stop the world and get off.

Danny Penman knows what he's talking about. His interest in meditation, taught to him briefly at school, was rekindled by an emergency. His paraglider failed and he fell from the sky. Badly injured, what could he do while waiting for the paramedics? He found his breath and, in an instant, everything changed. Then, in the long aftermath and months of recovery, what could he do to deal with the pain, the forced stillness, the boredom? What could he do in the face of the overwhelming thoughts about what had happened and the dreaded images of what might have happened if things had been even worse? He found his breath, again and again. It became a lifeline, a portal to a world of insight, of stability, and kindness. He had discovered mindfulness, the ancient wisdom of Asia, taught for two and a half thousand years. Mindfulness means clear-sighted, appreciative awareness. All of us are mindless sometimes and more aware at other times. And people differ, one from another, in the "set-point" of how much of the time they are mindful each day. But this set-point can be changed: both ancient wisdom and modern science show that mindful awareness can be cultivated by mental training.

I was privileged to get to know Danny when he, already an award-winning journalist writing on health, began to explore the research on mindfulness to see what others had discovered about it, and contacted me about the work that my colleagues and I were doing on how mindfulness could prevent serious clinical depression. Our research at Oxford was building on previous work done by Jon Kabat-Zinn, who had found that mindfulness reduced pain in those with chronic medical illness. Our research was showing that mindfulness training powerfully affects mental health, too. At times of great vulnerability, it prevents new episodes of depression from taking root, and even helps those who feel profoundly suicidal when depressed.

Danny suggested that we collaborate to take mindfulness out of the clinic and into the world, and the book *Mindfulness: A Practical Guide to Finding Peace in a Frantic World* was published in 2011. It showed that simple forms of meditation could be learned by anyone. Even a few weeks of paying sustained attention to what's going on from moment to moment, inside the mind and outside in the world, could have profound effects on the usual habits that tie you in knots and exhaust you. People all over the world began to find that when they learned how to pay attention moment by moment, intentionally and without judgment, they felt more at ease, more rested, less stressed, and spontaneously saw more of the small beauties and pleasures of the world they had taken for granted.

The path of learning mindfulness starts with the body. And this is where this book starts as well—with the simple act of noticing that you're breathing. The physical sensations that tell you that you are breathing have been with you since you were born, and you don't notice them most of the time—unless you suffer an illness that affects your breathing. Then you notice it. Then you realise that breath is life.

If you want to wake up to life as it is while you still can, beginning to sense the breath is a great start. But this book doesn't stop there. Eventually the steadiness that comes from allowing the breath to breathe itself allows you to see other things too. You come to see thoughts and emotions as if they were leaves on a stream or clouds in the sky, observing them as they come and go, without brooding about them or worrying about them. And so you have moved from the simple act of sensing the breath to the extraordinary insight that thoughts and feelings can be passing events if you allow them the space to arise and dissolve in consciousness. It's this ability to stand back a little and to see your thoughts and feelings clearly, which is at the heart of mindfulness. But it starts with the body, just as Danny says.

If you know a little about mindfulness, you may have read many similar descriptions of this practice. But what Danny Penman does in this book is not only offer the words but also set the words against images—leaves and branches, globe and cosmos—in which you cannot help but see the words emerging from and dissolving back into the natural world. And this itself invites us to let go of the urgency with which we often seek ways to reduce our stress (including the urgency to be mindful). It offers us a bigger time horizon—not clock time that entraps us, but horticultural time that sets everything in a wider context. The book does not just say "take your time," but it also shows us how to do so.

—Mark Williams
Emeritus Professor of Clinical Psychology,
University of Oxford

Acknowledgments

I am enormously grateful to Sheila Crowley at Curtis Brown. If you knew Sheila, you'd realize that she is quite simply the best agent and friend you could wish for. The same holds true for Kris Dahl of ICM Partners. She has done a great job of guiding my career in the US and Canada. And thanks to Lisa Milton of HQ. She mentioned the title of this book and everything fell into place. . . . She's one of those rare people who is full of brilliant ideas. When we're together, you can't shut either of us up. Thanks also to Greg Brandenburgh at Red Wheel/Weiser, who, together with Michael Pye, saw and then fell in love with *The Art of Breathing.* This US edition wouldn't have been possible without Christine LeBlond who edited this version. And thanks to Steve Wells who did the design and layout of this book. He's brilliant and I love his work.

Dr Danny Penman is a qualified meditation teacher and an award-winning writer and journalist. He is co-author of the international bestseller *Mindfulness: A Practical Guide to Finding Peace in a Frantic World*. He has received journalism awards from the RSPCA and the Humane Society of the United States. In 2014, he won the British Medical Association's Best Book (Popular Medicine) Award for *Mindfulness for Health: A Practical Guide to Relieving Pain, Reducing Stress and Restoring Wellbeing* (co-written with Vidyamala Burch). His books have been translated into thirty languages. His journalism has appeared in the *Daily Mail, New Scientist, The Independent, The Guardian,* and *The Daily Telegraph*. He trained to teach mindfulness with the acclaimed Breathworks.

HAMPTON ROADS
PUBLISHING COMPANY

... for the evolving human spirit

Hampton Roads Publishing Company publishes
books on a variety of subjects, including spirituality,
health, and other related topics.

For a copy of our latest trade catalog, call
(978) 465-0504 or visit our distributor's website at
www.redwheelweiser.com where you can also sign up
for our newsletter and special offers.